Safia OTHMANI
Hana HEDHLI
Rym BEN KADDOUR

Nursing management of critically ill patients in the ICU

Safia OTHMANI
Hana HEDHLI
Rym BEN KADDOUR

Nursing management of critically ill patients in the ICU

Role of the nurse in the management of patients in the emergency room

ScienciaScripts

Imprint

Any brand names and product names mentioned in this book are subject to trademark, brand or patent protection and are trademarks or registered trademarks of their respective holders. The use of brand names, product names, common names, trade names, product descriptions etc. even without a particular marking in this work is in no way to be construed to mean that such names may be regarded as unrestricted in respect of trademark and brand protection legislation and could thus be used by anyone.

Cover image: www.ingimage.com

This book is a translation from the original published under ISBN 978-620-3-42539-0.

Publisher:
Sciencia Scripts
is a trademark of
Dodo Books Indian Ocean Ltd., member of the OmniScriptum S.R.L Publishing group
str. A.Russo 15, of. 61, Chisinau-2068, Republic of Moldova Europe
Printed at: see last page
ISBN: 978-620-4-09864-7

Table of Contents

List of abbreviations

HMPIT: Main Military Hospital of Instruction of Tunis

HCN: Hôpital Charles Nicolle

SAUV: Emergency Room for Vital Emergencies

IDE : State qualified nurse

IAO: Reception and Orientation Nurse

ECG: Electrocardiogram

SAMU: Emergency Medical Service

SMUR : medical service

CP: Civil Protection

AED: Semi-automatic defibrillator

PPE: Personal Protective Equipment

VM : Mechanical ventilation

PISU: Emergency Care Nursing Protocols

DSI: Nursing Care Record

Introduction

Emergency departments are hospital services whose mission is to receive all people who are referred to them or who present themselves to them by ensuring that they are received and cared for appropriately according to their state of health. [1]

The number of patients admitted to emergency departments has been rising sharply in recent years, with nearly 21 million visits recorded in 641 public and private hospitals in 2016, 700,000 more than in 2015. [2]

This poses real problems for the management of vital emergencies that must receive urgent care. This is the reason for the creation of the so-called "Salles d'Accueil des Urgences Vitales" (SAUV), also known as dechoquage rooms, which constitute the hub of the emergency service, taking care of patients requiring an efficient and rapid intervention.

In 2003, a conference of experts from the French-speaking society of emergency medicine, the SAMU of France, the French society of anesthesia and resuscitation and the French-speaking resuscitation society was carried out to fill the absence of precise regulatory or legislative elements concerning the Salle d'Accueil des urgences vitales (SAUV). [3]

According to these recommendations, the SAUV is a place of reception which must be open 24 hours a day, does not correspond to a resuscitation bed or a hospitalization bed which must be released as soon as possible, and must be polyvalent and medico-surgical.

The proper functioning of such a unit depends on close collaboration between several stakeholders, of which the nurse plays an essential role with his or her own skills.

Nowadays, nurses have more and more responsibilities. They are on the front line of care and its organization, which makes this profession an important pillar in the quality of care.

During our time in the emergency department, we noticed that the nurse working in the UAS must master a set of technical and therapeutic procedures.

Thus, all caregivers must receive job adaptation training to be able to provide the necessary care in all sectors within the emergency department.

Indeed, the training of nurses allows them to identify medical emergencies, to practice gestures allowing them to provide assistance while waiting for the arrival of a medical team, to prioritize emergencies and to implement emergency care in a medical environment.

Dou our research questioning:

What is the role of the nurse in the management of patients in the ICU?

Hence we conducted a study that was interested in evaluating the attitudes of the nurse from the time of arrival until the completion of his work in the SAUV.

Materials andmethods

1- Location of the study

Our study took place in the emergency departments of the Charles Nicolle Hospital in Tunis (HCN) and the main military training hospital in Tunis (HMPIT). These services are polyvalent recording 125,000 passages per year.

Any patient, who presents with existing or potential vital distress, oriented from the triage by the reception and orientation nurse or arriving on a stretcher via the civil protection or the emergency medical service (SAMU) is admitted to the SAUV.

The SAUV must be well equipped with a rigorous organization to optimize the quality of care of serious cases that are life-threatening.

For this purpose, our shock room in the emergency department has the following elements:

- ➢ A ready-to-use emergency cart.
- ➢ An intubation tray.
- ➢ A scope with a central alarm system.
- ➢ A mobile lighting device.
- ➢ A defibrillator checked daily.
- ➢ A light box.
- ➢ Two modern respirators for invasive and non-invasive ventilation.
- ➢ Two manual suction devices.
- ➢ Two water points for hand washing.

The SAUV has a capacity of four simultaneous patients with three sliding curtains allowing to delimit the four care spaces four stations to condition the patients

Each station consists of :

- ➢ A stretcher bed adapted to resuscitation and patient transport.
- ➢ Two sockets for oxygen.
- ➢ An outlet for the air.
- ➢ Three sockets for the vacuum.
- ➢ A holder for monitoring devices and syringe pumps.

At each shift the nurse must make a checklist of all the material, check the functionality of all the devices, return all the equipment used after each intervention.

2- Type and period of the study :

We conducted a descriptive, observational, prospective study over a short period of time from March 15 to April 20.

3- Study population:

A. inclusion criteria:

The study population was composed of 40 nurses working frequently in SAUVs during all time slots (morning, afternoon and night).

B. Non-inclusion criteria :

Not included were:

-       Nurses practising in other departments other than emergency departments.

Nurses on leave.

- Trainees.

Nursing students

C. Exclusion criteria :

- Nurses who declined to participate in the study.

4- The data collection tool :

A. Observation grid :

We developed an observation grid to assess nurses' practices and attitudes and their role in the UAS.

We based our work on the latest expert conference of several learned societies on the establishment, management, use, and evaluation of a life-saving emergency room.

This observation grid analyzes the practices of the caregivers both during care and during the organization of this care: Passing between the nurses, the checklist, the acts of care provided for the patient.

Communication between team members: It is important to communicate and exchange information effectively between team members but also with the outside world.

B. Conduct of the study :

For the proper conduct of the study, the request for authorization was made to the heads of the emergency departments.

After consent was obtained, all participants were observed performing emergency procedures and care in their activities in the UAS.

We decided not to intervene so as not to bias the results of the study except for life-threatening behaviors.

5- Data management and analysis :

The data entry and the analysis of the results were done with the help of computer tools:

> Microsoft Office Word

> Microsoft Office Excel

The statistical analysis is presented in the form of graphs and tables.

6- Limitations of the study :

During our interview, we encountered some difficulties during the study:

- ✓ The coronavirus pandemic and the containment period hampered our work to collect a larger number of participants.
- ✓ The refusal of some nurses to participate in the study
- ✓ The time constraint.
- ✓ Nurses' compliance in the course of their work can influence their attitudes and change their behaviour.

7- Ethical consideration :

The data was collected in a way that respected the anonymity and confidentiality of the information.

We also declare the absence of conflicts of interest during the development of our work.

Results

I.   Demographic characteristics:

A total of 40 nurses were enrolled during the study period

1 Age:

The average age of the participants was 32 ±5 years with extremes from 24 to 41 years.

The distribution of participants shows a peak between the ages of 25 and 35.

Figure 1 shows the distribution of nurses by age group.

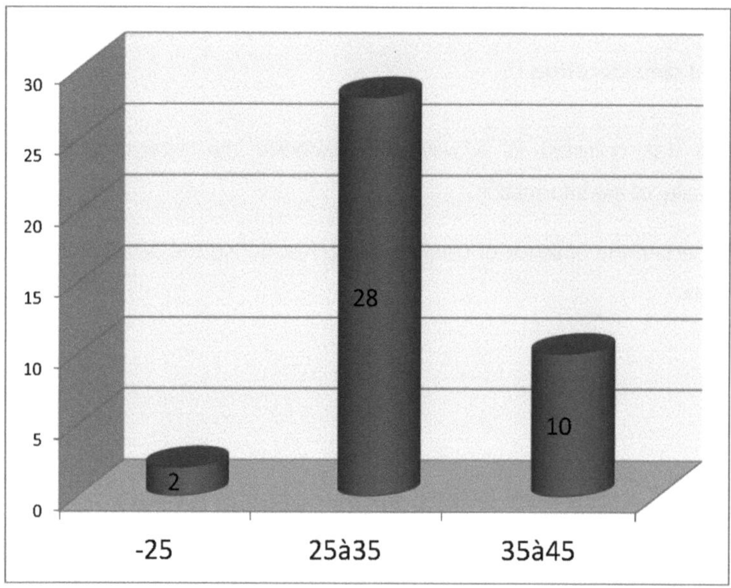

Figure 1: Distribution of nurses by age group

2. Gender:

There was a male predominance with a sex ratio of 1.22.

The following figure shows the distribution of participants by gender.

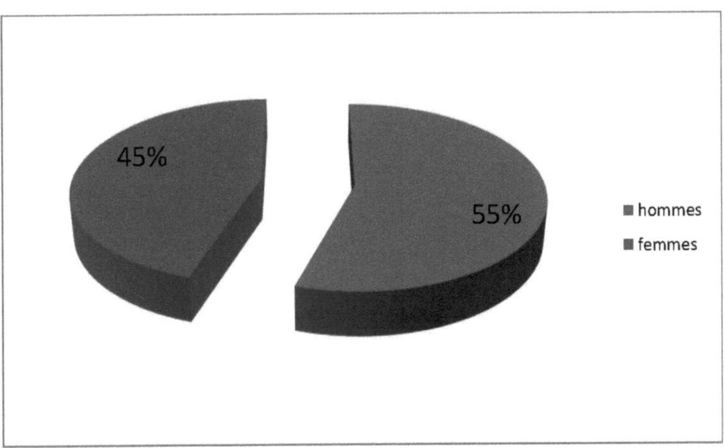

Figure 2: Distribution of nurses by gender

3. Academic training:

Our population consisted of 8 senior emergency medical technicians (20%) and 32 nurses (80%).

The following figure illustrates the distribution of participants by academic background:

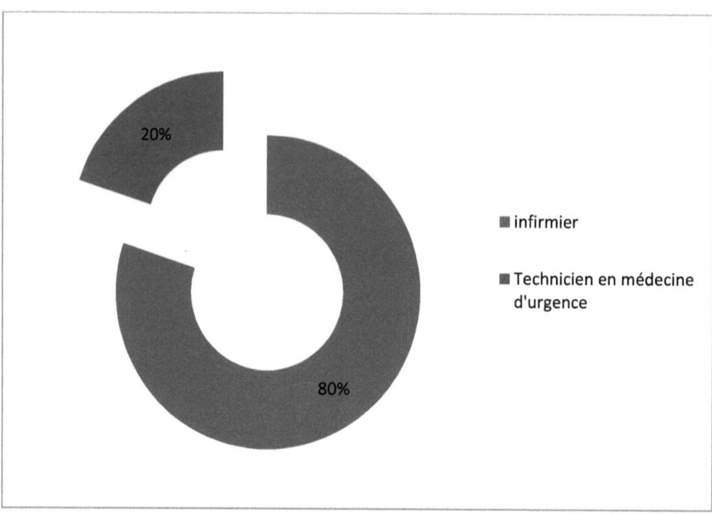

Figure 3: Distribution of nurses by academic background

4. Seniority in the service :

The majority of the participants have been working for 5 to 10 years and five people have been working for more than 10 years.

Figure 4 illustrates the distribution of nurses according to seniority in the department.

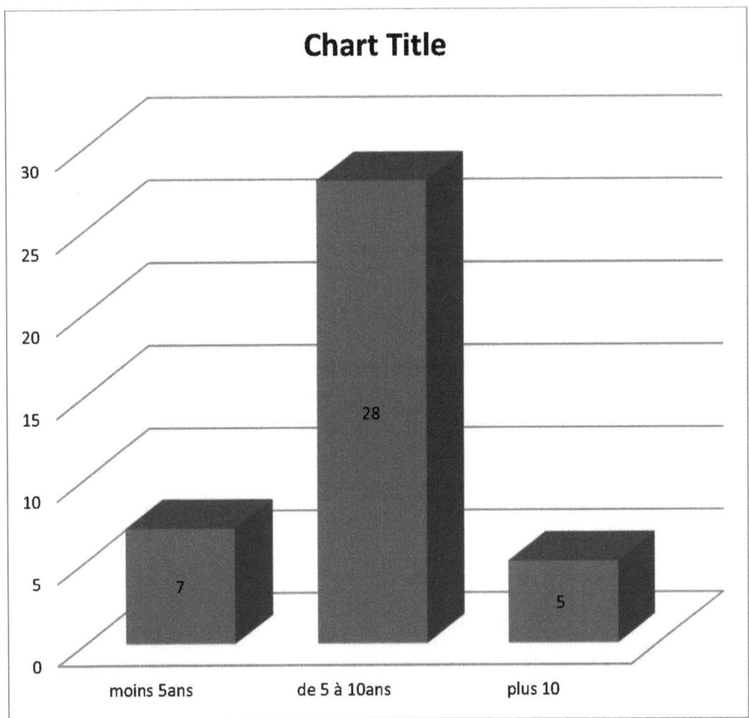

Figure 4: Distribution of nurses by length of service

II. Evaluation of nurses' attitudes

A. transmission of instructions :

Our study showed that the majority of participants (n=25, 62%) passed the instructions orally.

Communication between participants with clear and scientific language was noted in 67% of caregivers (n=27).

Seventy-five percent of the UAS nurses (n=30) informed their colleagues about the instructions not made.

Traceability on an instruction book was done by 55% of the participants.

Our study showed that 80% of the participants (n=32) work in collaboration.

No traceability of paramedical acts on a nursing file was found.

Table I summarizes nurses' attitudes about transmission between caregivers.

Table I: Distribution of nurses' attitudes regarding written and oral transmission.

Criteria	Values	N	(%)
Passing	written	15	37,5
	oral	25	62,5
Communication between staff with clear and scientific language	Yes	27	67,5
	No	13	32,5
Informing about a missed instruction	Yes	30	75
	No	10	25
Traceability in the form of a nursing file	Yes	0	0
	No	40	100
Traceability in the form of an instruction book	Yes	22	55
	No	18	45
Dynamic and collaborative teamwork	Yes	32	80
	No	8	20

B. Checklist :

Checking the emergency trolley was done by 82% of the nurses (n=33).

Fifteen participants (37%) prepared the intubation tray.

Eleven caregivers (27%) turned on the ventilators and performed the self-test.

Twenty-five percent of participants checked the room's defibrillator.

Seventy-two percent of nurses prepared the ECG machine.

The activation of the scopes of each bed was validated by all participants.

The table below shows the nurses' attitudes towards the checklist.

Table II: Nurses' attitudes towards the checklist

Criteria	Values	N	(%)
Checking the emergency trolley	Yes	33	82,5
	No	7	17,5
Preparation of the intubation tray	Yes	15	37,5
	No	25	62,5
Checking the suction system	Yes	27	67,5
	No	13	32,5
Switching on the respirators	Yes	11	27,5
	No	29	72,5
Defibrillator check	Yes	10	25
	No	30	75
Preparation of the ECG machine	Yes	29	72,5
	No	11	27,5
Switching on the scopes	Yes	40	100
	not	0	

C. Reception and care of patients:

Thirty-nine caregivers (98%) provided a welcome adapted to the patient's clinical condition upon arrival.

Sixty percent of the participants (n= 24) assessed the severity of the patients and determined the life-threatening emergency involved.

It was noted that 22.5% of the nurses (n=9) were able to assess the patient's pain using the appropriate scales for his or her condition

Five participants (12%) were interested in the patient's psychological state.

It was found that 27.5% (n=11) of the nurses performed the care on therapeutic protocols.

The majority of caregivers (n=3%) used personal protective equipment to reduce the risk of contamination.

Table III summarizes the distribution of nurses' attitudes regarding the reception and care of patients.

Table 1: The distribution of nurses' attitudes regarding the reception and care of patients.

Criteria	values	N	%
Specific reception adjusted according to the patient's condition on arrival	Yes	39	97,5
	No	1	2,5
Assess the patient's clinical condition and determine the degree of severity.	Yes	24	60
	No	16	40
Well oriented history according to the reason of hospitalization	Yes	22	55
	No	18	45
Patient identification	Yes	36	90
	No	4	10
Assessment of pain	Yes	9	22,5
	No	31	77,5

Assessment of the patient's psychological state	Yes	5	12,5
	No	35	87 ,5
Establish an empathetic relationship with the patient	Yes	24	60
	No	16	40
The implementation of care and therapy on protocol	Yes	11	27,5
	No	29	72,5
Follow and anticipate the evolution of the values of the monitoring parameters.	Yes	31	77,5
	No	9	22,5
Patient education	Yes	22	55
	No	18	45
Personal protection in case of suspected contagious disease	Yes	38	95
	No	2	5
Managing aggressive situations	Yes	16	40
	No	24	60

D. Relationship between staff

1. Work with mutual respect :

Eighty percent of the caregivers (n=32) in the SAUV work with mutual respect.

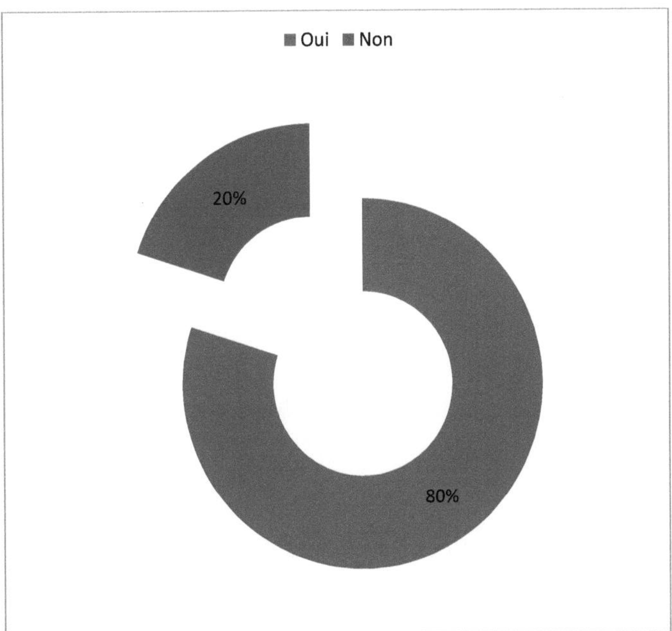

Figure 5: Distribution of nurses according to work in respect

2. Principle of Command and Principle of Authority :

Sixty-seven percent (n=27) of participants work with the command principle (LINE);

Thirty-three percent (n=13) of the participants work with the consulting authority principle (STAFF).

Figure 7 shows the distribution of nurses according to their work principles.

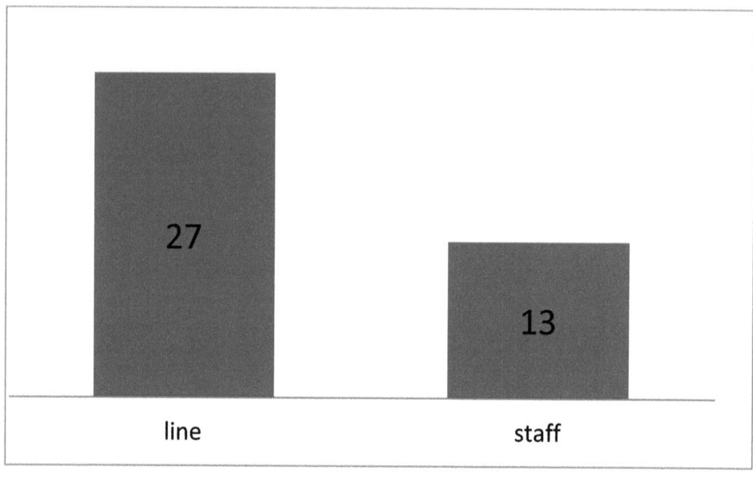

Figure 6: Principle of Command and Principle of Advisory Authority

Discussion

I.   Socio-demographic and professional criteria of the population :

The SAUV, or shock room, is a place where patients with existing or potential vital distress are received in the emergency department.

With the increase in the number of emergency department patients, the management of life-threatening conditions is becoming an increasing concern for emergency departments. [4]

For this, it requires a pre-established strategy for the organization of human and material resources in which the nurse plays a crucial role. [5]

In the light of this theme, our study was conducted to investigate the attitudes of nurses during the course of care in UVA.

To achieve our objective, we chose to proceed with a descriptive observational study through an observation grid intended for nurses working in the HMPIT and HCN emergency service.

Our population was young, with 70% of the participants aged between 25 and 35 years, and a male predominance was noted with a sex ratio of 1.22.

We noted that 80%(n=32) of the participants are nurses and 20%(n=8) are senior emergency medicine technicians, indeed the specialty in emergency medicine is a new branch which explains our results.

II. Transmission of instructions :

1- Oral and written transmissions :

The continuity of care depends on a good transmission of the instructions with exchange of information between the various intervening parties in the dechoking room.

In fact, the emergency room may have to deal unexpectedly with many victims requiring urgent resuscitation with continuous monitoring, therefore both written and oral transmission is a fundamental link in the chain of care for patients. [6]

Sixty-two percent of the participants (n=25) gave oral instructions to their colleagues and 37.5% (n=15) of the caregivers gave written instructions, with their actions recorded in an instruction booklet.

Seventy percent of participants were found to inform about the instructions not done.

It has been shown that oral transmission provokes immediate reactions by adapting to the person with possible readjustment of the content and, above all, allowing an exchange between the caregivers with a discussion that could be enriching for the management of the patients [7]. On the other hand, it allows to check the relevance and the understanding of the written information.

Nevertheless, oral transmission is fleeting, especially without any trace on the file, which can lead to forensic problems.

The receiver can be influenced by false perceptions, especially since verbal communication constitutes only 7% of the message transmitted. Thus, according to Albert Mehrebienthe body language is of decisive importance, because it is mainly what our interlocutor keeps in mind. [8]

At the same time, the oral transmission must be associated with a written transmission allowing to note all the actions of care carried out and to list all the observations and events which must be taken into account for their realization.

The written transmission is durable in time allowing a verification of the instructions at any moment of the care avoiding any omission. In addition, it engages the responsibility of the person who made it, thus making nurses much more vigilant. [9]

However, it is necessary to know how to choose the necessary and sufficient supports, adapted to the service, limited to essential and targeted information and avoiding secondary and uninteresting ones.

According to our study, caregivers communicate with each other in clear and scientific language in 67.5% (n=27) of cases.

In this context, Engouang L. et al [10] has shown that scientific language facilitates the work and the message between the different stakeholders. This must be clear, unambiguous and ensure that the information has been well assimilated by the receiver.

4- Traceability of the transmission

The emergency room is a dynamic place with many participants: nurses, emergency physicians, resuscitation anaesthetists, surgeons, SMUR team, civil protection team with, most of the time, background noise which can hinder the transmission of the message and facilitate misunderstandings. [11]

According to our study, it was noted that there is no nursing care record (NCR) for nurses to record instructions and actions performed.

The ISD is a personal document, customized for each patient, containing all the information concerning the person being cared for.

The ISD is not made mandatory by any text, but its constitution is highly recommended. [12]

Indeed, it has been introduced as a traceability support in the French context since 1970. It has undergone important evolutions over the last ten years. [13]

The aim of this file is to improve the quality of care (efficiency, continuity, safety) and the organization of care.

5- Dynamic and collaborative teamwork :

Eighty percent of participants (n= 32) work with dynamic teams.

The functions of each team member and their coordination to improve team performance in life-threatening emergencies is a quality factor that greatly influences the prognosis of patients admitted with a serious condition.

Thus, it has been demonstrated by a study made by Fabbrini et al [14] that good collaboration practices approved and respected by all team members are at the origin of cohesion and the development of mutual aid and constructive criticism.

III. Checklist

1- Checking the emergency trolley :

The majority of our population 82% (n=?) who work in the life-saving emergency room check the emergency cart at each shift. The participants check the emergency trolleys but in a quick and non-accurate way, which could expose to a delay in the management of extreme emergencies.

The emergency trolley is a fundamental element in the management of vital emergencies. It is under the responsibility of the nurse and the doctor assigned to the emergency room. [15]

In this context, it has been demonstrated by Reignier J et al [16] that the verification of the emergency tray is done according to a well determined procedure.

2- Preparation of the intubation tray :

Fifteen nurses (37%) prepared the intubation tray. This attitude of the nurses is explained by some caregivers that this task is considered a medical act. [17]

According to the recommendations of the French Society of Anaesthesia and Resuscitation, drugs and equipment for resuscitation of a patient in vital distress must be available immediately in order to reduce intervention times and facilitate management. [18]

3- Checking the suction system, starting up the respirators :

Twenty-seven caregivers (67.5%) checked the functionality of the suction system to ensure proper use when needed.

Eleven patients (27.5%) were able to handle the ventilators and ensure proper operation without leakage by self-testing.

In a multicentre study [19], involving 586 intensive care units in eight European countries, it was shown that the majority of decisions concerning MV are made in collaboration between the physician and the nurse.

According to our study, there were gaps and lack of skills regarding the procedures for checking and using ventilation machines, as well as maintenance and upkeep of the equipment. For paramedical staff, teaching emergency care with the use of equipment is an integral part of continuing education and a priority in the institution's training plan.

5- Checking the defibrillator, preparing the electrocardiogram:

The activation of the scopes was validated by all participants.

According to our study, we found 25% of the participants take the initiative to control the DSA and sometimes use it instead of a mobile scope.

Our study showed that 72.5% of the participants prepare the machine and perform an ECG when needed or when prescribed by a doctor.

Indeed, the majority of health care personnel working in emergency departments do not check the functionality of the defibrillator upon arrival at the department.

It has been demonstrated in article 5 of the decree of nursing competence that "the nurse is entitled to perform on written, qualitative and quantitative, dated and signed medical prescription, nursing acts or care provided that a doctor can intervene at any time, among these acts we found the use of a semi-automatic defibrillator and monitoring of the patient placed under this device [20].

The performance of an ECG is a nursing act on medical delegation. However, the nurse takes the initiative to perform an emergency ECG for patients presenting to the emergency department with chest pain and present it to a qualified person for interpretation within 10 minutes. [21]

IV. Home :

1- Specific reception adjusted according to the patient's condition on arrival

It was noted that a specific reception adjusted according to the patient's condition on arrival is validated by all the participants.

The emergency department is a transitional service, and as a result, the main part of the nurse-patient relationship in the emergency department is the reception of the patient. Despite the multifactorial difficulties mentioned, it is important for both partners that this first contact is not trivialized. As M. Formarier [23] points out, "the reception is a complex professional act that is crucial for the rest of the relationship".

Hence we found that our participants do a quick sort for each new admission which is recommended by MASSON E. [24]

2- Assess the patient's clinical condition and determine the degree of severity:

Twenty-four of the participants (60%) assessed the clinical severity of patients with a well-directed history by reason for hospitalization (n=22, (55%).

Thus, the orientation and intake nurse (IOA) must be able to collect and analyze a range of clinical data and alert the physician to any signs of severity that require immediate medical intervention[25].

Thus Cloutier L et al [26] emphasized the importance of a thorough history of the patient and his entourage in order to orient the patient to the sector best suited to his care.

5- Assessment of pain and psychological state of the patient :

Nine participants assessed the patient's pain and five caregivers were interested in the patient's psychological state.

Pain is the fourth vital distress after respiratory, hemodynamic and neurological distress and its treatment is urgently required.

The assessment of pain intensity is the first step in pain management. For this purpose, several tools have been proposed, including self-evaluation and hetero-evaluation. Self-evaluation concerns communicating patients and hetero-evaluation concerns non-communicating patients. The quality of the management depends on the quality of the assessment. [27]

7- Establish an empathic relationship with the patient:

Our study showed that 60% of the caregivers (n=24) established an empathic relationship with their patients according to their reasons for admission.

It has been found that creating an empathic relationship with the patient greatly assists nurses to better perform their care and improve patient response to treatment.

According to Robin et al [28], these activities are important to optimize patient management by adopting active listening and minimizing tension in the emergency room.

8- Care provided on protocol :

In emergency departments and in case of admission of a patient in vital distress in the UAS, it has been noticed that sometimes there is no doctor in these critical situations. However, nurses must intervene immediately to try to save the patient's life.

Our study showed that only 27.5% of the nurses implement the care according to precise protocols previously established.

Following the circular concerning the implementation of the reference system for the organization of the emergency medical assistance service, the French Society of Emergency Medicine (SFMU), together with the French learned societies, has elaborated nursing care protocols, called emergency care nursing protocols (PISU) for the clinical situations that can be the subject of the initiation of these protocols by the nurses. [29]

Our participants do not find protocols to follow when performing their procedures in the life-saving emergency room.

9- Follow and anticipate the evolution of the values of the monitoring parameters:

It was noted that 77.5% (n=31) of the health care personnel follow and anticipate the evolution of the values of the monitoring parameters.

The monitoring of the patients received in the vital emergency rooms is a primary task that must be done by the nurse working in this position.

The rhythm of patient monitoring depends on the clinical condition of the patient, and according to the study by BARON et al [30], vital parameters such as blood pressure, respiratory rate, heart rate, temperature and oxygen saturation are the responsibility of the nurses.

10- Patient education :

Fifty-five percent of the participants (n=22) opted for patient education by giving advice about their chronic diseases to prevent complications and acute decompensation.

According to Karin et al, patient education is an integral part of care. [31]

Furthermore, it was noted that patient education is a concept that is not well understood by health professionals.

Therefore, we propose to integrate patient education into the training of health professionals.

11- Personal protection in case of suspected contagious disease :

Our study was developed in a period of pandemic (COVID-19) and therefore, it was noted that all staff working in emergency departments wore all the PPE to minimize the risk of contamination and this according to the recommendations of the National Authority for Health Evaluation and Accreditation (INEAS). [32]

12- Managing aggressive situations :

Sixty percent of the participants (n=24) were unable to manage and control aggressive situations by patients received in emergency departments or by attendants.

Our results are similar with those of Ferrari et al [33] who showed that in 2012, 350 health facilities had more than 8,000 reports of violence to persons.

The prevention of these aggressive acts consists in improving the reception and the conditions of stay in the emergency room, reducing the waiting time of the patients and improving the information of the patients and the accompanying persons with a reliable and clear communication in order to build a relation of confidence with them.

V. Relationship between staff :

1- Working with mutual respect :

Our study showed that the work and relationship between the staff was in mutual respect with 80% (n=32) of the caregivers trying to solve the problems and find suitable solutions despite the work stress and congestion of the SAUV.

2- Principle of command (line) and Principle of advisory authority (staff) :

According to our study, 68%(n=27) of the nurses stated that the principle of work in the emergency life support room is the principle of command and 32.5%(n=13) of the teams prefer the principle of advisory authority.

Line is the principle of unity of command and scale of authority. Thus, the line provides for a hierarchical authority which is nothing other than the translation of the authority relationship between a manager and his subordinates.

Hence, this principle was found generally in the reception room of vital emergencies of the main military hospital of instruction of Tunis given the military ranks.

The principle of the line consists of three components:

1. Command (a leader).

2. Leadership (a totality of actions with a single objective and a single leader).

3. The centralization of the unit (this is the pyramidal hierarchy). [34]

Staff is the principle of a supreme authority who is there to chaperone the line managers. In other words, the staff is the management team.

While the staff advises the managers, it should be noted that it does not have to explain the consequences of its decisions. The staff plays the role of functional authority.

This principle was found in the Charles Nicolle hospital.

VI. Recommendations

The nurse, in collaboration with the whole team of the care service, is on the front line to act in an emergency situation. He is often the referent of the team while waiting for the arrival of the doctor. The nurse must therefore be able to deal with emergency situations of the patients he will be in charge of in the care unit where he will practice. [35]

In light of the results of this study, many gaps in nursing practice and quality of care were revealed, leading us to propose the following recommendations:

- ➢ Each patient arriving in the SAUV must have a nursing file to ensure the traceability of nursing acts.
- ➢ Organization of training for emergency nurses to improve nursing skills and care qualities to better deal with unscheduled cases. Nurses working in emergency departments must be senior technicians in emergency medicine.
- ➢ Precise and pre-established protocols for the emergency nurse to welcome the patient, assess his or her state of gravity and even administer medication and medical procedures according to standards in case of the doctor's absence.
- ➢ Training in health communication techniques: the emergency nurse must be able to communicate (with colleagues, patients, patient's family), to persuade others in order to determine his tasks and also to manage aggressive situations and to ensure the education of his patients.
- ➢ Educate the teams working in the SAUVs on the principles and concepts of teamwork and provide LEADERSHIP training for the team leader.

Conclusions

The idea for this thesis began with the observation of gaps and practices that diverge from the recommendations in the PACU where we did our internship for 3 months. Our objective was to evaluate the attitudes of the caregivers by observing the different tasks performed by the nurse and his reactions with the patients and the colleagues in the outpatient department.

The results of this research allowed us to make a professional reflection aiming at making us project our professional future.

Indeed, we had many preconceived ideas about the realities of the nursing profession. During the three years of training, we realized that most of our preconceived ideas were in fact false and that the daily professional practice was related to an incalculable number of problems that sometimes seem far from the real practices of nurses.

Our study consists of an observation and evaluation study of nursing acts in the SAUV within the emergency services of HMPIT and HCN of Tunis.

The nurse's actions were divided into 4 main items: Reception, Checklist, Interpersonal relations and Passing of instructions.

The results showed us that there are knowledge gaps that can affect the quality of work.

It was found that most instructions were given orally. In addition, we did not find a nursing record under the responsibility of the nurse for each patient.

The nursing acts during the reception of a patient are not totally in accordance with the recommendations, so the assessment of pain was underestimated, although it is a crucial step in the management of patients.

The implementation of care protocols in the emergency department allows to prioritize and plan the care activities according to the parameters of the context and the urgency of the situations.

From our study it was found that there were no pre-established protocols to guide the assessment and emergency management of patients when the physician was not immediately available.

Hence, recommendations were proposed to improve work in emergency rooms. The need for training for nurses working in this type of context must be considered in order to reassure future practitioners.

References

1. Guide pour la mise en place de procédures de prise en charge d'un patient aux urgences, République Tunisienne ministère de la santé, Direction générale de la santé. Circular N 81/2005 2003

2. ANNE BAYLE-INIGUEZ, Le quotidien médecin, 26/06/2018 Available at: lequotidiendumedecin.fr

3. Recommendations concerning the implementation, management, use and evaluation of a life-saving emergency room (L.E.R.) Page Société Francophone de Médecine d'Urgencehttp://www.sfmu.orgMise à Journee définitive Février 2003

4. Carrasco B. Emergency room users: first results of a national survey. 2003;8.

5. Recommendations for the establishment, management, use, and evaluation of a life-saving emergency room (LER). Resuscitation. March 2004;13(2):154 8

6. GOUIN Simon: Analysis of the use of the Emergency Room

Vitals of the Hospital Center of Pau. Doctoral thesis.2016

7. Transmissions [Internet]. IDE Guide. 2018 [cited June 17, 2020]. Available from: https://guide-ide.com/les-transmissions/

8. Collins, Amy Lee; Jordan, Peter; Troth, AshleaThe impact of team emotional intelligence on team affect, conflict and performance: a preliminary analysis. British Academy of Management ConferenceProceedings 2014.

9. MACSF.fr. The nurse facing an oral prescription - MACSF [Internet]. MACSF.fr. [cited 17 June 2020]. Available from: https://www.macsf.fr/Responsabilite-professionnelle/Actes-de-soins-et-technique-medicale/infirmier-prescription-orale

10. Engouang L-SO. Translation between teaching tool and scientific discipline: the case of Spanish in Gabon and Equatorial Guinea. :527

11. Fatima-Zahra Lkharrat. Management of organizational problems in the vital emergency room. Thesis for the degree of Doctor of Medicine. 2019

12. Brunet O. DSI 2020: deadline for the social declaration of the self-employed [Internet]. Practical life. 2019 [cited 17 June 2020]. Available from: https://www.toutsurmesfinances.com/vie-pratique/a/dsi-date-limite-de-la-declaration-sociale-des-independants

13. The computerized nursing record [Internet]. [cited June 17, 2020]. Available from: https://www.caducee.net/DossierSpecialises/systeme-information-sante/dsii.asp

14. Fabbrini H. How to make teamwork a performance lever? [Internet]. [cited 17 June 2020]. Available from: https://blog.monportailrh.com/6-astuces-pour-faire-du-travail-en-equipe-un-puissant-levier-pour-la-performance

15. Decree No. 2002-194 of 11 February 2002 on the professional acts and practice of the profession of nursing. 2002-194 Feb. 11, 2002

16. REIGNIER J., PROCEDURE DE VÉRIFICATION ET DE MAINTENANCE DES CHARIOTS D'URGENCE, 1 :4]

17. Baillard C, Fosse JP, Sebbane M, Chanques G, Vincent F, Courouble P, Cohen Y, Eledjam JJ, Adnet F, Jaber S : Noninvasive ventilation improves preoxygenation before intubation of hypoxic patients. Am J Respir Crit Care Med 2006; 174: 171-7

18. French Society of Anesthesia and Intensive Care. 2004]

19. Netgen. Nurse-physician collaboration: a determinant of quality of care? [Internet]. Swiss Medical Journal. [cited 17 June 2020]. Available from: https://www.revmed.ch/RMS/2005/RMS-42/30804

20. Decree 93-345 of 15 March 1993 on the professional acts and practice of the profession of nurse (known as the decree on nursing competence)

21. French Society of Emergency Medicine, nurse outside medical presence, page 4

22. Patrick K. 2016 - Electrocardiogram. :75

23. Formarier M. APPROACHING THE CONCEPT OF HOME, BETWEEN BANALITY AND COMPLEXITY. 2003;6.

24. Masson E. The role of the nurse organizer in the emergency room [Internet]. EM-Consult. [cited June 17, 2020]. Available from: https://www.em-consulte.com/article/659630/le-role-de-linfirmiere-organisateur-de-laccueil-au

25. Boursin P, Maillard-Acker C. L'examen clinique infirmier, un outil de l'IOA (Infirmier Organisateur de l'Accueil). :10

26. Cloutier L. La pratique infirmière de l'examen clinique. De Boeck 2010 : 389 p.)

27. Galinski M, Adnet F. Management of acute pain in emergency medicine. Reanimation. nov 2007;16(7 8):652 9.]

28. Robin-Quach P. Knowing the patient's representations to optimize the educational project. Nursing research. 2009;N° 98(3):36 68

29. Pateron D. PROFESSIONAL RECOMMENDATIONS. 2015;15.

30. DESMETTRE T, BARON AF, CAPELLIEr G, Tazarourte K. The nurse reception organizer (NRI): role and functions. Réanimation. Nov 2013;22(6):610 5

31. Karin van Balleko, patient education in hospitals February 2008

32. New coronavirus (2019-nCoV): advice to the general public [Internet]. [cited 18 June 2020]. Available from: https://www.who.int/fr/emergencies/diseases/novel-coronavirus-2019/advice-for-public]

33. Ferrari R. Violence in the emergency room: a sad reality? :9.

34. Management course - What is the staff and line structure? [Internet]. [cited 18 June 2020]. Available from: https://www.pimido.com/blog/vie-etudiant/cours-management-ce-structure-staff-line-06-03-2018.html

35. Dumas M, Douguet F, Fahmi Y. The good functioning of care services: what makes a team? RIMHE: Revue Interdisciplinaire Management, Homme Entreprise. 2 Feb 2016;No. 20(1):45 67

ANNEXS
Annex I

Role of the nurse in the emergency room

Data collection form

The nurse : XY   Age :   years old

Gender: Male   ☐   Female   ☐

Married   ☐   Single ☐

Year of graduation: Emergency technician   ☐ Multi-skilled nurse ☐

Seniority in the job: Seniority in the emergency department:

Role of the nurse in patient care in the UAS			
Role of the nurse	**Yes**	**No**	**Remarks**
Home			
Specific reception adjusted according to the patient's condition on arrival			
Assess the patient's clinical condition and determine the degree of severity.			
Well oriented history according to the reason of hospitalization			
Patient identification			
Assessment of pain			
Assessment of the patient's psychological state			
Establish an empathetic relationship with the patient			
The implementation of care and therapy on protocol			
Follow and anticipate the evolution of the values of the monitoring parameters.			
Patient education			
Personal protection in case of suspected contagious disease			
Managing aggressive situations			
checklist			
Checking the emergency trolley			
Preparation of the intubation tray			
Checking the suction system			
Switching on the respirators			
Defibrillator check			
Preparation of the electrocardiogram machine			
Switching on the scopes			
Relationship between staff			
Work with mutual respect			
Principle of command (line)			

Principle of advisory authority (staff)			
Passing of instructions			
Oral test			
Written test			
Communication between staff with clear and scientific language			
Informing about a missed instruction			
Traceability in the form of a nursing file			
Traceability in the form of an instruction book			
Dynamic and collaborative teamwork			

ANNEX II

ECHELLE VISUELLE ANALOGIQUE (EVA): Face présentée au patient

Pas de douleur   Douleur maximale imaginable

Recto : face graduée en millimètres de 0 à 100.

ECHELLE NUMERIQUE (EN)

Echelle quantitative de 0 à 10 : « Donnez une note à votre douleur de 0 à 10 ».

ECHELLE VERBALE SIMPLE (EVS)

- Chaque descripteur associé à une valeur numérique

    0 = Pas de douleur

    1 = Faible

    2 = Modérée

    3 = Intense

    4 = Atroce

ANNEX III

ALGOPLUS

Echelle d'évaluation comportementale de la douleur aiguë

chez la personne âgée présentant des troubles de la communication verbale

	Oui	Non
1 – Visage : **Froncement des sourcils, grimaces, crispation, mâchoires serrées, visage figé**	☐	☐
2 – Regard : **Regard inattentif, fixe, lointain ou suppliant, pleurs, yeux fermés**	☐	☐
3 – Plaintes orales : **« Aie », « Ouille », « j'ai mal », gémissements, cris**	☐	☐
4 – Corps : **Retrait ou protection d'une zone, refus de mobilisation, attitudes figées**	☐	☐
5 – Comportements : **Agitation ou agressivité, agrippement**	☐	☐

Total : Oui |___| / 5

Title: The role of the nurse in the management of patients in emergency rooms

Summary

Introduction: Emergency departments receive patients whose vital prognosis is at stake. They are admitted to the Vital Emergency Room. The proper functioning of such a unit depends on the collaboration between several stakeholders, of which the nurse plays a key role with his own skills. The objective of our study was to evaluate the practice of the nurse from his arrival until the completion of his work in the SAUV.

Methods: This is a descriptive, prospective, observational study carried out in the emergency department of the Military Hospital of Tunis and Charles Nicolle Hospital. An observation grid was developed with 4 main items to describe and evaluate the skills of nurses in the SAUV.

Results: Our population consisted of 40 participants divided into 32 nurses and 8 emergency medicine technicians. The average age was 32±5 years. The transmission of instructions was done orally in 62% of the cases. Thus, we did not find a nursing care file and we noted that traceability was done in the form of an instruction book used by 55% of the participants. The verification of the intubation tray was carried out in 82% of the cases, whereas the intubation tray and the defibrillator were only checked in 37% and 25% respectively. Pain assessment was underestimated. The reception and care provided were satisfactory in most cases. An empathetic relationship with the patients and a mutual respect between the different members of the team were noted.

Conclusion: Our study revealed shortcomings in the attitudes of nurses in the emergency room, which led us to propose recommendations for improving the behaviour of caregivers.

More
Books!

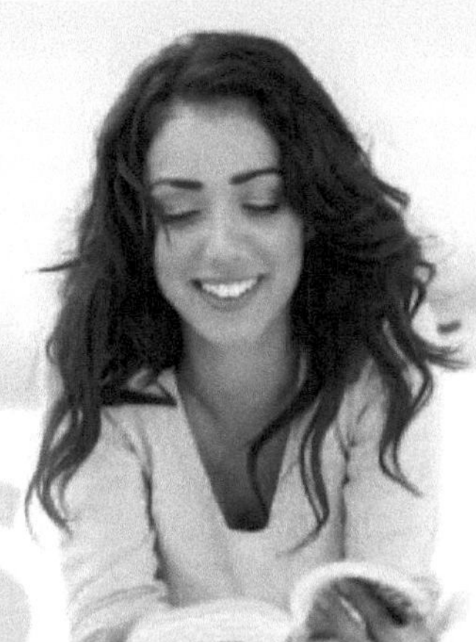

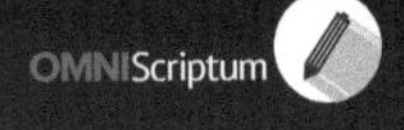

OMNIScriptum

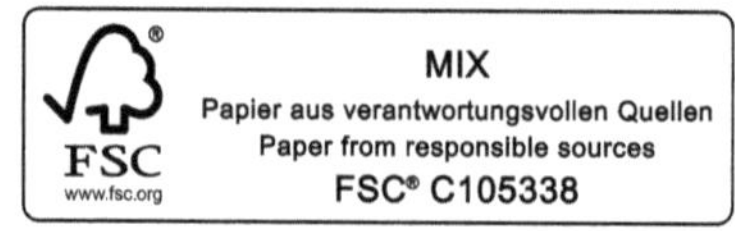

Printed by Books on Demand GmbH, Norderstedt / Germany